DIABETIC-FRIENDLY PLANT-BASED RECIPES FOR BEGINNERS

Delicious and easy-to-follow diabetic-friendly plant-based recipes for beginners, perfect for managing blood sugar levels and improving your overall health.

Dr Lily Morgan

COPYRIGHT PAGE

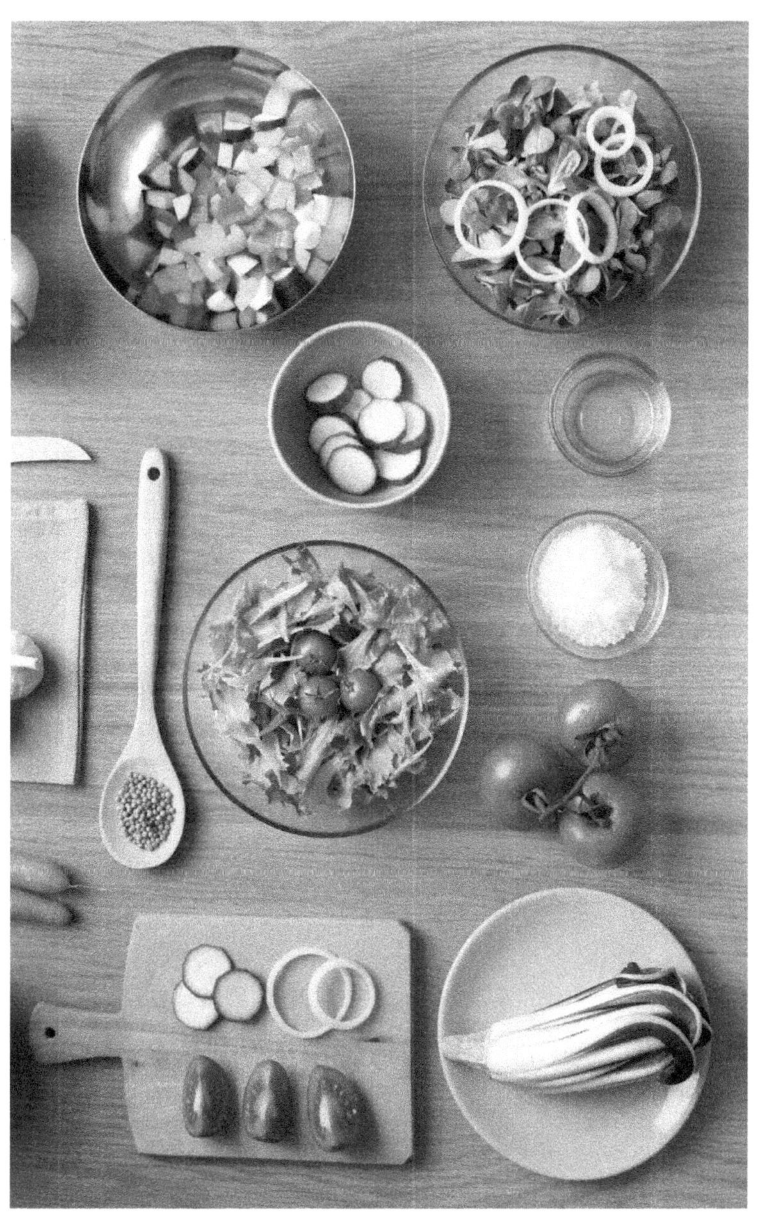

TABLE OF CONTENTS

Chapter 6: Desserts 90

INTRODUCTION

I n the world of health and nutrition, one topic that has gained considerable attention is the relationship between diabetes and plant-based diets. To grasp this connection, we need to first comprehend the intricacies of diabetes.

Diabetes is a chronic condition characterized by elevated levels of blood sugar, often caused by the body's inability to produce or properly utilize insulin. There are two main types of diabetes: Type 1 and Type 2. Type 1 diabetes is an autoimmune condition where the body's immune system mistakenly attacks and destroys the insulin-producing cells in the pancreas. Type 2 diabetes, on the other hand, is primarily linked to lifestyle factors, such as poor diet and lack of physical activity, which can lead to insulin resistance and an inadequate insulin response.

The role of diet in managing diabetes cannot be overstated. It is here that plant-based diets come into focus. A plant-based diet emphasizes the consumption of foods derived from plants, including vegetables, fruits, grains, legumes, nuts, and seeds, while minimizing or eliminating animal products. This dietary approach is characterized by its potential to positively influence diabetes management and prevention.

Benefits of a Diabetic-Friendly Plant-Based Diet

1. **Improved Blood Sugar Control:** Plant-based diets, rich in fiber, complex carbohydrates, and low in saturated fats, can help regulate blood sugar levels. Fiber slows down the absorption of glucose, preventing rapid spikes, and providing steady energy throughout the day.

2. **Weight Management:** Maintaining a healthy weight is essential for individuals with diabetes. Plant-based diets are often lower in calories and saturated fats, making it easier to manage and lose weight, which can improve insulin sensitivity.

3. **Heart Health:** Cardiovascular issues are a significant concern for people with diabetes. Plant-based diets are associated with lower cholesterol

levels, reduced blood pressure, and a decreased risk of heart disease, offering a protective shield for the heart.

4. **Lower Risk of Complications:** By reducing inflammation and oxidative stress, a plant-based diet can lower the risk of diabetes-related complications, such as nerve damage, kidney disease, and eye problems.

5. **Versatile Food Choices:** A plant-based diet is incredibly diverse, allowing for a wide range of flavors, textures, and culinary experiences. This makes it more appealing and sustainable for individuals managing diabetes.

6. **Enhanced Insulin Sensitivity**: Some research suggests that a plant-based diet may improve insulin sensitivity, making it easier for the body to utilize insulin effectively.

In summary, understanding the synergy between diabetes and plant-based diets is pivotal for those seeking to take control of their health and well-being. By adopting a diabetic-friendly plant-based diet, individuals can experience a multitude of benefits, from better blood sugar control to improved overall health. It's not just a dietary choice; it's a pathway to a healthier, more vibrant life.

Chapter 1: 30-Day Meal Plan

Week 1:

Day 1:

- Breakfast: Oatmeal with Fresh Berries
- Lunch: Chickpea Salad
- Dinner: Ratatouille
- Snacks: Guacamole with Veggie Sticks
- Dessert: Banana Ice Cream

Day 2:

- Breakfast: Avocado Toast with a Twist
- Lunch: Spinach and Strawberry Salad
- Dinner: Stuffed Bell Peppers
- Snacks: Salsa and Baked Tortilla Chips
- Dessert: Vegan Chocolate Avocado Mousse

Day 3:

- Breakfast: Chia Seed Pudding
- Lunch: Quinoa and Black Bean Bowl
- Dinner: Mushroom Risotto

- Snacks: Edamame with Sea Salt
- Dessert: Berry Parfait

Day 4:

- Breakfast: Veggie Breakfast Burrito
- Lunch: Lentil Soup
- Dinner: Black Bean and Sweet Potato Stew
- Snacks: Carrot and Cucumber Slices with Hummus
- Dessert: Coconut Bliss Balls

Day 5:

- Breakfast: Vegan Pancakes
- Lunch: Greek Couscous Salad
- Dinner: Vegan Chili
- Snacks: Vegan Spring Rolls
- Dessert: Chia Seed Pudding with Berries

Day 6:

- Breakfast: Fruit and Nut Smoothie
- Lunch: Veggie Wrap with Hummus
- Dinner: Spaghetti Squash with Tomato Sauce
- Snacks: Roasted Red Pepper Hummus

- Dessert: Vegan Chocolate Chip Cookies

Day 7:

- Breakfast: Quinoa Porridge
- Lunch: Tomato Basil Bruschetta
- Dinner: Thai Green Curry
- Snacks: Avocado Fries
- Dessert: Almond Joy Energy Bites

Week 2:

Day 8:

- Breakfast: Breakfast Tofu Scramble
- Lunch: Sweet Potato and Black Bean Tacos
- Dinner: Eggplant Parmesan
- Snacks: Sweet Potato Fries
- Dessert: Vegan Apple Crisp

Day 9:

- Breakfast: Sweet Potato Hash
- Lunch: Grilled Portobello Mushrooms
- Dinner: Baked Tofu with Teriyaki Glaze
- Snacks: Stuffed Mushrooms

- Dessert: Chocolate-Dipped Strawberries

Day 10:

- Breakfast: Breakfast Muffins
- Lunch: Asian-Inspired Noodle Salad
- Dinner: Quinoa-Stuffed Acorn Squash
- Snacks: Quinoa-Stuffed Bell Peppers
- Dessert: Cinnamon Baked Apples

Day 11:

- Breakfast: Spinach and Mushroom Quiche
- Lunch: Cauliflower Buffalo Bites
- Dinner: Moroccan Lentil Stew
- Snacks: Vegan Onion Rings
- Dessert: Vegan Rice Pudding

Day 12:

- Breakfast: Peanut Butter Banana Sandwich
- Lunch: Caprese Salad
- Dinner: Portobello Steaks
- Snacks: Roasted Chickpeas
- Dessert: Mango Sorbet

Day 13:

- Breakfast: Zucchini Fritters
- Lunch: Spinach and Lentil Soup
- Dinner: Vegan Alfredo Pasta
- Snacks: Vegan Spinach Artichoke Dip
- Dessert: Vegan Pumpkin Pie

Day 14:

- Breakfast: Overnight Muesli
- Lunch: Roasted Vegetable Sandwich
- Dinner: Butternut Squash and Kale Salad
- Snacks: Cucumber Avocado Rolls
- Dessert: Chocolate Zucchini Brownies

Week 3:

Day 15:

- Breakfast: Vegan French Toast
- Lunch: Soba Noodle Salad
- Dinner: Mediterranean Stuffed Zucchini
- Snacks: Stuffed Grape Leaves
- Dessert: Lemon Blueberry Bars

Day 16:

- Breakfast: Blueberry Buckwheat Pancakes
- Lunch: Vegan Caesar Salad
- Dinner: Vegan Jambalaya
- Snacks: Baked Zucchini Chips
- Dessert: Vegan Cheesecake

Day 17:

- Breakfast: Green Smoothie Bowl
- Lunch: Roasted Red Pepper and Chickpea Wraps
- Dinner: Cauliflower Steaks
- Snacks: Vegan Bruschetta
- Dessert: Berry Sorbet

Day 18:

- Breakfast: Mexican Breakfast Bowl
- Lunch: Chickpea Salad
- Dinner: Ratatouille
- Snacks: Guacamole with Veggie Sticks
- Dessert: Banana Ice Cream

Day 19:

- Breakfast: Avocado Toast with a Twist
- Lunch: Spinach and Strawberry Salad
- Dinner: Stuffed Bell Peppers
- Snacks: Salsa and Baked Tortilla Chips
- Dessert: Vegan Chocolate Avocado Mousse

Day 20:

- Breakfast: Chia Seed Pudding
- Lunch: Quinoa and Black Bean Bowl
- Dinner: Mushroom Risotto
- Snacks: Edamame with Sea Salt
- Dessert: Berry Parfait

Day 21:

- Breakfast: Veggie Breakfast Burrito
- Lunch: Lentil Soup
- Dinner: Black Bean and Sweet Potato Stew
- Snacks: Carrot and Cucumber Slices with Hummus
- Dessert: Coconut Bliss Balls

Week 4:

Day 22:

- Breakfast: Mexican Breakfast Bowl
- Lunch: Chickpea Salad
- Dinner: Ratatouille
- Snacks: Guacamole with Veggie Sticks
- Dessert: Banana Ice Cream

Day 23:

- Breakfast: Oatmeal with Fresh Berries
- Lunch: Spinach and Strawberry Salad
- Dinner: Stuffed Bell Peppers
- Snacks: Salsa and Baked Tortilla Chips
- Dessert: Vegan Chocolate Avocado Mousse

Day 24:

- Breakfast: Avocado Toast with a Twist
- Lunch: Quinoa and Black Bean Bowl
- Dinner: Mushroom Risotto
- Snacks: Edamame with Sea Salt
- Dessert: Berry Parfait

Day 25:

- Breakfast: Chia Seed Pudding
- Lunch: Lentil Soup
- Dinner: Black Bean and Sweet Potato Stew
- Snacks: Carrot and Cucumber Slices with Hummus
- Dessert: Coconut Bliss Balls

Day 26:

- Breakfast: Veggie Breakfast Burrito
- Lunch: Greek Couscous Salad
- Dinner: Vegan Chili
- Snacks: Vegan Spring Rolls
- Dessert: Chia Seed Pudding with Berries

Day 27:

- Breakfast: Fruit and Nut Smoothie
- Lunch: Veggie Wrap with Hummus
- Dinner: Spaghetti Squash with Tomato Sauce
- Snacks: Roasted Red Pepper Hummus
- Dessert: Vegan Chocolate Chip Cookies

Day 28:

- Breakfast: Quinoa Porridge
- Lunch: Tomato Basil Bruschetta
- Dinner: Thai Green Curry
- Snacks: Avocado Fries
- Dessert: Almond Joy Energy Bites

Day 29:

- Breakfast: Breakfast Tofu Scramble
- Lunch: Sweet Potato and Black Bean Tacos
- Dinner: Eggplant Parmesan
- Snacks: Sweet Potato Fries
- Dessert: Vegan Apple Crisp

Day 30:

- Breakfast: Sweet Potato Hash
- Lunch: Grilled Portobello Mushrooms
- Dinner: Baked Tofu with Teriyaki Glaze
- Snacks: Stuffed Mushrooms
- Dessert: Chocolate-Dipped Strawberries

This plan covers a full 30 days, providing you with a variety of diabetic-friendly, plant-based meals for beginners to enjoy. You can continue to repeat this cycle for a longer period if needed.

Chapter 2: Breakfast Recipes

Welcome to the breakfast section of our diabetic-friendly plant-based cookbook. Mornings are a time to kickstart your day with energy and flavor while keeping your health in mind. These breakfast recipes are designed to do just that – they are not only delicious but also perfect for maintaining a balanced diet while managing diabetes.

Oatmeal with Fresh Berries

Ingredients:

- 1/2 cup rolled oats
- 1 cup almond milk
- 1/4 cup fresh mixed berries (strawberries, blueberries, raspberries)
- 1 tablespoon chia seeds
- 1 tablespoon honey or maple syrup (optional)

Instructions:

1. In a saucepan, bring almond milk to a simmer.

2. Stir in the rolled oats and cook until they reach your desired consistency.

3. Transfer to a bowl, top with fresh berries and chia seeds.

4. Drizzle with honey or maple syrup if desired.

Avocado Toast with a Twist

Ingredients:

- 2 slices of whole-grain bread
- 1 ripe avocado
- 1 small tomato, sliced
- 1/4 red onion, thinly sliced
- Fresh basil leaves
- Salt and pepper to taste

Instructions:

1. Toast the bread until crispy.

2. Mash the ripe avocado and spread it on the toasted slices.

3. Top with tomato slices, red onion, and fresh basil.

4. Season with salt and pepper to taste.

Chia Seed Pudding

Ingredients:

- 3 tablespoons chia seeds
- 1 cup almond milk
- 1/2 teaspoon vanilla extract
- Fresh mixed berries for topping

Instructions:

1. Mix chia seeds, almond milk, and vanilla extract in a jar or bowl.
2. Refrigerate for at least 2 hours or overnight.
3. Before serving, stir the mixture, and top with fresh mixed berries.

Veggie Breakfast Burrito

Ingredients:

- 1 whole-grain tortilla
- 1/2 cup cooked quinoa
- 1/4 cup black beans
- 1/4 cup sautéed bell peppers and onions
- Salsa or hot sauce (optional)

Instructions:

1. Lay the tortilla flat and add quinoa, black beans, and sautéed bell peppers and onions.
2. Roll it up, tucking in the sides.
3. Heat on a skillet to warm and crisp the tortilla.
4. Serve with salsa or hot sauce if desired.

Vegan Pancakes

Ingredients:

- 1 cup whole wheat flour
- 1 tablespoon baking powder
- 1 tablespoon sugar
- 1 cup almond milk
- 2 tablespoons applesauce
- 1 teaspoon vanilla extract

Instructions:

1. In a bowl, whisk together flour, baking powder, and sugar.
2. Add almond milk, applesauce, and vanilla extract, and mix until well combined.
3. Heat a non-stick skillet over medium-high heat.

4. Pour 1/4 cup of batter for each pancake and cook until bubbles form on top.

5. Flip and cook until golden brown.

Fruit and Nut Smoothie

Ingredients:

- 1 cup spinach
- 1/2 banana
- 1/2 cup mixed berries
- 1 tablespoon almond butter
- 1 cup almond milk

Instructions:

1. Add spinach, banana, mixed berries, and almond butter to a blender.
2. Pour in almond milk.
3. Blend until smooth and creamy.

Quinoa Porridge

Ingredients:

- 1/2 cup quinoa

- 1 cup almond milk
- 1/4 teaspoon cinnamon
- 1/4 cup sliced almonds
- Fresh fruit for topping

Instructions:

1. Rinse quinoa thoroughly.
2. In a saucepan, combine quinoa, almond milk, and cinnamon.
3. Bring to a simmer, then reduce heat and cover.
4. Cook for about 15 minutes until quinoa is tender.
5. Serve with sliced almonds and fresh fruit on top.

Breakfast Tofu Scramble

Ingredients:

- 1/2 block of firm tofu, crumbled
- 1/4 cup diced bell peppers
- 1/4 cup diced onions
- 1/4 cup spinach
- 1/2 teaspoon turmeric
- Salt and pepper to taste

Instructions:

1. In a skillet, sauté bell peppers and onions until softened.
2. Add crumbled tofu and turmeric, cook for 3-5 minutes.
3. Add spinach and cook until wilted.
4. Season with salt and pepper.

Sweet Potato Hash

Ingredients:

- 1 medium sweet potato, diced
- 1/4 cup diced bell peppers
- 1/4 cup diced onions
- 1/4 cup black beans
- 1/2 teaspoon paprika
- Salt and pepper to taste

Instructions:

1. In a skillet, sauté sweet potatoes, bell peppers, and onions until tender.
2. Add black beans, paprika, salt, and pepper.
3. Cook for a few more minutes until heated through.

Breakfast Muffins

Ingredients:

- 1 cup whole wheat flour
- 1/4 cup rolled oats
- 1/4 cup raisins or dried cranberries
- 1/4 cup chopped nuts
- 1 teaspoon baking powder
- 1/4 cup maple syrup
- 1/2 cup almond milk

Instructions:

1. Preheat your oven to 350°F (175°C) and line a muffin tin with paper liners.
2. In a bowl, mix the flour, oats, raisins or cranberries, nuts, and baking powder.
3. In another bowl, combine the maple syrup and almond milk.
4. Pour the wet ingredients into the dry ingredients and stir until just combined.
5. Spoon the batter into the muffin cups and bake for about 20-25 minutes, or until a toothpick comes out clean.

Spinach and Mushroom Quiche

Ingredients:

- 1 pre-made whole wheat pie crust
- 1 cup spinach, chopped
- 1 cup mushrooms, sliced
- 1/2 cup diced onions
- 1 cup tofu, crumbled
- 1/4 cup almond milk
- 1/2 teaspoon turmeric
- Salt and pepper to taste

Instructions:

1. Preheat your oven to 375°F (190°C).
2. Sauté mushrooms and onions until soft.
3. In a separate bowl, mix crumbled tofu, almond milk, turmeric, salt, and pepper.
4. Add spinach, mushrooms, and onions to the tofu mixture.
5. Pour the mixture into the pie crust and bake for 30-35 minutes until set.

Peanut Butter Banana Sandwich

Ingredients:

- 2 slices of whole-grain bread
- 2 tablespoons peanut butter
- 1 banana, sliced

Instructions:

1. Spread peanut butter on one slice of bread.
2. Arrange banana slices on top.
3. Top with the second slice of bread.

Zucchini Fritters

Ingredients:

- 2 zucchinis, grated
- 1/4 cup whole wheat flour
- 1/4 cup nutritional yeast
- 1/2 teaspoon garlic powder
- Salt and pepper to taste
- 1 flax egg (1 tablespoon ground flaxseed mixed with 3 tablespoons water)
- Olive oil for frying

Instructions:

1. In a bowl, combine grated zucchini, whole wheat flour, nutritional yeast, garlic powder, salt, and pepper.
2. Mix in the flax egg.
3. Heat olive oil in a skillet over medium heat.
4. Form the mixture into patties and cook until golden brown on both sides.

Overnight Muesli

Ingredients:

*   1/2 cup rolled oats
*   1/2 cup almond milk
*   1/4 cup Greek yogurt
*   1/4 cup mixed berries
*   1 tablespoon honey or maple syrup (optional)

Instructions:

1. Combine rolled oats, almond milk, and Greek yogurt in a jar or bowl.
2. Refrigerate overnight.

3. Top with mixed berries and drizzle with honey or
   maple syrup if desired.

Vegan French Toast

Ingredients:

- 2 slices of whole-grain bread
- 1/4 cup almond milk
- 1 tablespoon chickpea flour
- 1/2 teaspoon vanilla extract
- 1/2 teaspoon cinnamon
- Maple syrup and fresh fruit for topping

Instructions:

1. In a bowl, whisk together almond milk, chickpea
   flour, vanilla extract, and cinnamon.
2. Dip the bread slices in the mixture, ensuring they are
   coated.
3. Cook in a skillet until golden brown on both sides.
4. Serve with maple syrup and fresh fruit.

Blueberry Buckwheat Pancakes

Ingredients:

- 1 cup buckwheat flour
- 1 teaspoon baking powder
- 1/4 teaspoon salt
- 1 cup almond milk
- 1/2 cup fresh blueberries
- 1 tablespoon maple syrup

Instructions:

1. In a bowl, combine buckwheat flour, baking powder, and salt.
2. Add almond milk and mix until smooth.
3. Gently fold in fresh blueberries.
4. Cook small pancakes on a hot skillet until they bubble on top, then flip and cook until golden brown.
5. Drizzle with maple syrup.

Green Smoothie Bowl

Ingredients:

- 1 cup spinach

- 1/2 banana

- 1/2 cup pineapple chunks

- 1/2 cup almond milk

- Toppings: sliced almonds, chia seeds, fresh fruit

Instructions:

1. Blend spinach, banana, pineapple, and almond milk until smooth.

2. Pour into a bowl and top with sliced almonds, chia seeds, and fresh fruit.

Mexican Breakfast Bowl

Ingredients:

- 1/2 cup cooked quinoa

- 1/4 cup black beans

- 1/4 cup corn

- 1/4 cup diced tomatoes

- 1/4 avocado, sliced

- Salsa and hot sauce (optional)

Instructions:

1. Combine cooked quinoa, black beans, corn, and diced tomatoes in a bowl.

2. Top with avocado slices.

3. Add salsa and hot sauce for an extra kick if desired.

Chapter 3: Lunch Recipes

In this chapter, we'll explore a delightful array of lunchtime options that are not only delicious but also perfect for those looking to maintain a diabetic-friendly plant-based diet. These recipes are thoughtfully crafted to tantalize your taste buds while keeping your health in mind. From vibrant salads to hearty soups and satisfying wraps, you'll find an assortment of flavors and textures to enjoy.

Chickpea Salad

Ingredients:

- 2 cups canned chickpeas, drained and rinsed
- 1 cucumber, diced
- 1 red bell pepper, chopped
- 1/4 cup red onion, finely chopped
- 1/4 cup fresh parsley, chopped
- 2 tablespoons olive oil
- 1 lemon, juiced
- Salt and pepper to taste

Instructions:

1. In a large bowl, combine chickpeas, cucumber, red bell pepper, red onion, and parsley.
2. Drizzle with olive oil and lemon juice.
3. Season with salt and pepper.
4. Toss gently to mix, and your chickpea salad is ready to serve.

Spinach and Strawberry Salad

Ingredients:

- 4 cups fresh spinach leaves
- 1 cup sliced strawberries
- 1/4 cup slivered almonds
- 2 tablespoons balsamic vinaigrette dressing
- 1 tablespoon agave nectar

Instructions:

1. In a salad bowl, combine spinach, strawberries, and slivered almonds.
2. Drizzle with balsamic vinaigrette dressing and agave nectar.

3. Toss to coat, and your spinach and strawberry salad is ready to enjoy.

Quinoa and Black Bean Bowl

Ingredients:

- 1 cup cooked quinoa
- 1 cup black beans, drained and rinsed
- 1 cup corn kernels
- 1/2 red onion, finely chopped
- 1/4 cup fresh cilantro, chopped
- 2 tablespoons lime juice
- 1 teaspoon cumin
- Salt and pepper to taste

Instructions:

1. In a bowl, combine cooked quinoa, black beans, corn, red onion, and cilantro.
2. In a separate bowl, whisk together lime juice, cumin, salt, and pepper.
3. Pour the dressing over the quinoa mixture and toss to combine.

Lentil Soup

Ingredients:

- 1 cup dried green or brown lentils
- 1 carrot, chopped
- 1 celery stalk, chopped
- 1 onion, finely chopped
- 2 cloves garlic, minced
- 6 cups vegetable broth
- 1 teaspoon cumin
- 1/2 teaspoon paprika
- Salt and pepper to taste

Instructions:

1. In a large pot, sauté onion, garlic, carrot, and celery until softened.
2. Add lentils, vegetable broth, cumin, paprika, salt, and pepper.
3. Simmer for about 30 minutes or until the lentils are tender.

Greek Couscous Salad

Ingredients:

- 1 cup cooked couscous
- 1 cucumber, diced
- 1 tomato, chopped
- 1/4 cup Kalamata olives, pitted and sliced
- 1/4 cup red onion, finely chopped
- 1/4 cup feta cheese, crumbled
- 2 tablespoons olive oil
- 1 tablespoon lemon juice
- Fresh oregano leaves (optional)

Instructions:

1. In a large bowl, combine cooked couscous, cucumber, tomato, Kalamata olives, red onion, and feta cheese.
2. Drizzle with olive oil and lemon juice.
3. Toss gently and garnish with fresh oregano leaves, if desired.

Veggie Wrap with Hummus

Ingredients:

- Whole wheat tortillas
- 1 cup hummus
- Assorted vegetables (e.g., bell peppers, carrots, cucumber)
- Spinach leaves

Instructions:

1. Spread a generous layer of hummus on a whole wheat tortilla.
2. Layer on your choice of assorted vegetables and spinach leaves.
3. Roll up the tortilla tightly, and your veggie wrap with hummus is ready to be savored.

Tomato Basil Bruschetta

Ingredients:

- 4 ripe tomatoes, diced
- 1/4 cup fresh basil leaves, chopped
- 2 cloves garlic, minced

- 2 tablespoons olive oil
- Salt and pepper to taste
- Whole grain baguette slices

Instructions:

1. In a bowl, combine diced tomatoes, fresh basil, garlic, and olive oil.
2. Season with salt and pepper.
3. Serve the tomato basil mixture on whole grain baguette slices.

Sweet Potato and Black Bean Tacos

Ingredients:

- 2 medium sweet potatoes, peeled and cubed
- 1 can black beans, drained and rinsed
- 1 teaspoon cumin
- 1/2 teaspoon chili powder
- Whole wheat tortillas
- Avocado slices
- Salsa

Instructions:

1. Roast sweet potato cubes with cumin and chili powder until tender.

2. Warm whole wheat tortillas and fill them with roasted sweet potatoes, black beans, avocado slices, and salsa.

Grilled Portobello Mushrooms

Ingredients:

- Portobello mushrooms
- Balsamic vinegar
- Olive oil
- Garlic powder
- Salt and pepper

Instructions:

1. Marinate Portobello mushrooms in a mixture of balsamic vinegar, olive oil, garlic powder, salt, and pepper.

2. Grill until tender and serve as a healthy, savory dish.

Asian-Inspired Noodle Salad

Ingredients:

- Whole wheat noodles
- Cucumber, julienned
- Carrots, julienned
- Edamame beans
- Sesame seeds
- Soy ginger dressing

Instructions:

1. Cook whole wheat noodles according to package instructions.
2. Toss the cooked noodles with cucumber, carrots, and edamame beans.
3. Drizzle with soy ginger dressing and sprinkle with sesame seeds.

Cauliflower Buffalo Bites

Ingredients:

- Cauliflower florets
- Buffalo sauce (vegan)

- Olive oil

- Garlic powder

- Dipping sauce (vegan ranch or hummus)

Instructions:

1. Toss cauliflower florets in a mixture of buffalo sauce, olive oil, and garlic powder.

2. Bake until crispy and serve with your choice of dipping sauce.

Caprese Salad

Ingredients:

- Tomatoes, sliced

- Fresh mozzarella, sliced

- Fresh basil leaves

- Balsamic glaze

- Olive oil

- Salt and pepper

Instructions:

1. Arrange alternating slices of tomatoes, fresh mozzarella, and fresh basil on a plate.

2. Drizzle with balsamic glaze and olive oil.

3. Season with salt and pepper for a classic Caprese salad.

Spinach and Lentil Soup

Ingredients:

- 1 cup dried green or brown lentils
- 1 carrot, chopped
- 1 celery stalk, chopped
- 1 onion, finely chopped
- 2 cloves garlic, minced
- 6 cups vegetable broth
- 2 cups fresh spinach leaves
- 1 teaspoon cumin
- 1/2 teaspoon paprika
- Salt and pepper to taste

Instructions:

1. In a large pot, sauté onion, garlic, carrot, and celery until softened.

2. Add lentils, vegetable broth, cumin, paprika, salt, and pepper.

3. Simmer for about 30 minutes or until the lentils are
   tender.
4. Stir in fresh spinach leaves just before serving.

Roasted Vegetable Sandwich

Ingredients:

- Whole grain bread
- Roasted vegetables (e.g., bell peppers, zucchini,
  eggplant)
- Hummus
- Fresh basil leaves

Instructions:

1. Spread hummus on slices of whole grain bread.
2. Layer with roasted vegetables and fresh basil leaves
   for a satisfying sandwich.

Spinach and Walnut Pesto Pasta

Ingredients:

- Whole wheat pasta
- Fresh spinach leaves

- Walnuts

- Garlic cloves

- Olive oil

- Nutritional yeast (optional)

- Salt and pepper

Instructions:

1. Blend fresh spinach, walnuts, garlic, olive oil, and nutritional yeast (if desired) into a pesto sauce.

2. Toss with cooked whole wheat pasta, and season with salt and pepper.

Soba Noodle Salad

Ingredients:

- Soba noodles

- Cucumber, julienned

- Carrots, julienned

- Edamame beans

- Sesame seeds

- Soy ginger dressing

Instructions:

1. Cook soba noodles according to package instructions.
2. Toss the cooked noodles with cucumber, carrots, and edamame beans.
3. Drizzle with soy ginger dressing and sprinkle with sesame seeds.

Vegan Caesar Salad

Ingredients:

- Romaine lettuce, chopped
- Vegan Caesar dressing
- Croutons (whole grain if possible)
- Vegan Parmesan cheese (optional)

Instructions:

1. Toss chopped Romaine lettuce with vegan Caesar dressing.
2. Top with croutons and vegan Parmesan cheese, if desired.

Roasted Red Pepper and Chickpea Wraps

Ingredients:

- Whole wheat tortillas
- Roasted red peppers
- Chickpeas, mashed
- Spinach leaves
- Tahini sauce

Instructions:

1. Spread mashed chickpeas on whole wheat tortillas.
2. Layer with roasted red peppers, spinach leaves, and drizzle with tahini sauce.
3. Roll up the wraps, and they're ready to enjoy.

Chapter 4: Dinner Recipes

In this chapter. These recipes are not only healthy but also rich in flavors that will satisfy your taste buds. Whether you're a fan of traditional favorites or you're in the mood to explore new culinary horizons, this collection has something for everyone. Let's dive into these delectable dinner recipes that are sure to become a staple in your plant-based repertoire.

Ratatouille

Ingredients:

- 1 eggplant, sliced
- 2 zucchinis, sliced
- 2 red bell peppers, sliced
- 1 onion, chopped
- 3 cloves of garlic, minced
- 4 tomatoes, diced
- 2 tablespoons olive oil
- 1 teaspoon dried thyme
- 1 teaspoon dried basil

- Salt and pepper to taste

Instructions:

1. Preheat your oven to 375°F (190°C).
2. In a large baking dish, layer the eggplant, zucchini, and bell peppers.
3. In a separate pan, sauté the onion and garlic in olive oil until translucent.
4. Add tomatoes, thyme, basil, salt, and pepper to the pan. Cook for a few minutes.
5. Pour the tomato mixture over the layered vegetables.
6. Cover the baking dish with foil and bake for 45 minutes. Then, uncover and bake for an additional 15 minutes until the vegetables are tender.

Stuffed Bell Peppers

Ingredients:

- 4 bell peppers, any color
- 1 cup cooked quinoa
- 1 can black beans, drained and rinsed
- 1 cup corn kernels
- 1 cup diced tomatoes

- 1/2 cup diced onion
- 1 teaspoon chili powder
- 1/2 teaspoon cumin
- Salt and pepper to taste
- 1 cup tomato sauce

Instructions:

1. Preheat the oven to 350°F (175°C).
2. Cut the tops off the bell peppers and remove seeds.
3. In a bowl, mix cooked quinoa, black beans, corn, diced tomatoes, onion, chili powder, cumin, salt, and pepper.
4. Stuff each bell pepper with the mixture.
5. Place the stuffed peppers in a baking dish, pour tomato sauce over them.
6. Cover with foil and bake for 30-35 minutes until peppers are tender.

Mushroom Risotto

Ingredients:

- 1 cup Arborio rice
- 2 cups vegetable broth

- 1 cup mushrooms, sliced
- 1/2 cup onion, chopped
- 2 cloves garlic, minced
- 1/2 cup white wine
- 2 tablespoons olive oil
- 1/4 cup nutritional yeast (optional)
- Salt and pepper to taste

Instructions:

1. In a saucepan, heat olive oil and sauté onions and garlic until translucent.
2. Add Arborio rice and stir for a couple of minutes.
3. Pour in white wine and stir until absorbed.
4. Gradually add vegetable broth, one ladle at a time, stirring constantly until absorbed.
5. Stir in sliced mushrooms and nutritional yeast.
6. Continue adding broth and stirring until the rice is creamy and tender.
7. Season with salt and pepper.

Black Bean and Sweet Potato Stew

Ingredients:

- 2 cups sweet potatoes, diced
- 2 cups black beans, cooked
- 1 onion, chopped
- 3 cloves garlic, minced
- 1 red bell pepper, diced
- 1 can diced tomatoes
- 4 cups vegetable broth
- 2 teaspoons chili powder
- 1 teaspoon cumin
- Salt and pepper to taste

Instructions:

1. In a large pot, sauté onions and garlic until fragrant.
2. Add sweet potatoes, black beans, red bell pepper, diced tomatoes, vegetable broth, chili powder, cumin, salt, and pepper.
3. Simmer for about 20-25 minutes until sweet potatoes are tender.
4. Serve hot.

Vegan Chili

Ingredients:

- 1 can black beans, drained and rinsed
- 1 can kidney beans, drained and rinsed
- 1 can diced tomatoes
- 1 cup corn kernels
- 1 onion, chopped
- 2 cloves garlic, minced
- 2 tablespoons chili powder
- 1 teaspoon cumin
- 1/2 teaspoon paprika
- Salt and pepper to taste

Instructions:

1. In a large pot, sauté onions and garlic until translucent.
2. Add black beans, kidney beans, diced tomatoes, corn, chili powder, cumin, paprika, salt, and pepper.
3. Simmer for about 20-25 minutes, stirring occasionally.

Spaghetti Squash with Tomato Sauce

Ingredients:

- 1 spaghetti squash
- 2 cups tomato sauce (homemade or store-bought)
- 1 tablespoon olive oil
- 2 cloves garlic, minced
- 1/2 teaspoon dried basil
- 1/2 teaspoon dried oregano
- Salt and pepper to taste

Instructions:

1. Preheat the oven to 375°F (190°C).
2. Cut the spaghetti squash in half, remove the seeds, and drizzle with olive oil.
3. Place the squash halves cut side down on a baking sheet and bake for 35-45 minutes until the flesh is tender.
4. Meanwhile, in a saucepan, heat the olive oil and sauté garlic until fragrant.
5. Add tomato sauce, basil, oregano, salt, and pepper. Simmer for a few minutes.

6. Scrape the cooked spaghetti squash with a fork to create "noodles" and serve with tomato sauce.

Thai Green Curry

Ingredients:

- 1 can coconut milk
- 2 tablespoons green curry paste
- 1 cup mixed vegetables (e.g., bell peppers, broccoli, carrots)
- 1 cup tofu, cubed
- 1 tablespoon soy sauce
- 1 tablespoon brown sugar
- Fresh basil leaves
- Cooked rice or noodles for serving

Instructions:

1. In a large pan, heat the coconut milk and green curry paste over medium heat.
2. Add mixed vegetables and tofu.
3. Stir in soy sauce and brown sugar. Simmer until the vegetables are tender and the tofu is heated through.
4. Serve with fresh basil leaves over rice or noodles.

Eggplant Parmesan

Ingredients:

- 2 large eggplants, sliced
- 2 cups marinara sauce
- 1 cup breadcrumbs (use gluten-free if needed)
- 1/2 cup vegan Parmesan cheese
- 2 teaspoons dried basil
- 2 teaspoons dried oregano
- Salt and pepper to taste
- Olive oil for frying

Instructions:

1. Dip eggplant slices in marinara sauce, then coat with breadcrumbs, vegan Parmesan, basil, oregano, salt, and pepper.
2. Heat olive oil in a skillet and fry the coated eggplant slices until golden brown.
3. Place the fried eggplant in a baking dish, layer with marinara sauce, and bake at 375°F (190°C) for 25-30 minutes until bubbly.

Baked Tofu with Teriyaki Glaze

Ingredients:

- 1 block tofu, pressed and cubed
- 1/2 cup teriyaki sauce (make sure it's vegan)
- 1 tablespoon sesame seeds
- Sliced green onions for garnish

Instructions:

1. Preheat the oven to 375°F (190°C).
2. Marinate tofu cubes in teriyaki sauce for about 15 minutes.
3. Place marinated tofu on a baking sheet and sprinkle with sesame seeds.
4. Bake for 20-25 minutes, turning tofu halfway through.
5. Garnish with sliced green onions.

Quinoa-Stuffed Acorn Squash

Ingredients:

- 2 acorn squashes, halved and seeds removed
- 1 cup quinoa, cooked

- 1 cup mixed vegetables (e.g., bell peppers, zucchini, carrots)
- 1/2 cup dried cranberries
- 1/4 cup chopped pecans
- 1 tablespoon olive oil
- 1 teaspoon dried thyme
- Salt and pepper to taste

Instructions:

1. Preheat the oven to 375°F (190°C).
2. Brush the acorn squash halves with olive oil, season with salt and pepper, and place them on a baking sheet.
3. In a bowl, mix cooked quinoa, mixed vegetables, dried cranberries, chopped pecans, dried thyme, salt, and pepper.
4. Stuff each squash half with the quinoa mixture.
5. Bake for 40-45 minutes or until the squash is tender.

Moroccan Lentil Stew

Ingredients:

- 1 cup green or brown lentils, rinsed

- 1 onion, chopped
- 3 cloves garlic, minced
- 1 carrot, diced
- 1 zucchini, diced
- 1 can diced tomatoes
- 4 cups vegetable broth
- 2 teaspoons ground cumin
- 1 teaspoon ground coriander
- 1/2 teaspoon ground cinnamon
- Salt and pepper to taste

Instructions:

1. In a large pot, sauté onions and garlic until translucent.
2. Add lentils, carrot, zucchini, diced tomatoes, vegetable broth, cumin, coriander, cinnamon, salt, and pepper.
3. Simmer for about 25-30 minutes until lentils and vegetables are tender.

Portobello Steaks

Ingredients:

- 4 large Portobello mushrooms
- 1/4 cup balsamic vinegar
- 2 tablespoons olive oil
- 2 cloves garlic, minced
- 1 teaspoon dried rosemary
- Salt and pepper to taste

Instructions:

1. Clean Portobello mushrooms and remove the stems.
2. In a bowl, mix balsamic vinegar, olive oil, garlic, rosemary, salt, and pepper.
3. Marinate mushrooms in the mixture for about 30 minutes.
4. Grill or bake the mushrooms for 10-12 minutes on each side.

Vegan Alfredo Pasta

Ingredients:

- 8 oz fettuccine pasta (use gluten-free if needed)

- 1 cup cauliflower florets
- 1/2 cup cashews, soaked and drained
- 2 cloves garlic
- 1/2 cup almond milk
- 2 tablespoons nutritional yeast
- 1 tablespoon lemon juice
- Salt and pepper to taste

Instructions:

1. Cook fettuccine pasta according to package instructions.
2. Steam cauliflower until tender.
3. In a blender, combine cauliflower, soaked cashews, garlic, almond milk, nutritional yeast, lemon juice, salt, and pepper.
4. Blend until smooth.
5. Toss the cooked pasta with the Alfredo sauce and serve.

Butternut Squash and Kale Salad

Ingredients:

- 4 cups butternut squash, diced

- 4 cups kale, chopped
- 1/4 cup dried cranberries
- 1/4 cup pumpkin seeds
- 2 tablespoons olive oil
- 1 tablespoon balsamic vinegar
- Salt and pepper to taste

Instructions:

1. Preheat the oven to 375°F (190°C).
2. Toss butternut squash with olive oil, salt, and pepper.
3. Roast the squash for 20-25 minutes until tender.
4. In a bowl, massage kale with balsamic vinegar until it wilts slightly.
5. Toss roasted butternut squash, dried cranberries, and pumpkin seeds with the kale.

Mediterranean Stuffed Zucchini

Ingredients:

- 4 zucchinis
- 1 cup cooked quinoa
- 1/2 cup cherry tomatoes, halved
- 1/2 cup Kalamata olives, chopped

- 1/4 cup red onion, finely chopped
- 2 cloves garlic, minced
- 2 tablespoons olive oil
- 1 teaspoon dried oregano
- Salt and pepper to taste

Instructions:

1. Preheat the oven to 375°F (190°C).
2. Cut zucchinis in half lengthwise and scoop out the centers.
3. In a bowl, mix cooked quinoa, cherry tomatoes, Kalamata olives, red onion, garlic, olive oil, dried oregano, salt, and pepper.
4. Stuff the zucchini halves with the quinoa mixture.
5. Bake for 20-25 minutes until zucchini is tender.

Vegan Jambalaya

Ingredients:

- 1 cup brown rice
- 1 cup vegetable broth
- 1 onion, chopped
- 1 green bell pepper, diced

- 1 celery stalk, diced

- 2 cloves garlic, minced

- 1 can kidney beans, drained and rinsed

- 1 can diced tomatoes

- 2 teaspoons Cajun seasoning

- 1/2 teaspoon paprika

- Salt and pepper to taste

Instructions:

1. In a large pot, sauté onions, green bell pepper, celery, and garlic until translucent.

2. Add brown rice and vegetable broth.

3. Stir in kidney beans, diced tomatoes, Cajun seasoning, paprika, salt, and pepper.

4. Simmer for about 25-30 minutes until rice is cooked.

Cauliflower Steaks

Ingredients:

- 2 large cauliflower heads

- 2 tablespoons olive oil

- 1 teaspoon smoked paprika

- 1/2 teaspoon garlic powder

- 1/2 teaspoon onion powder
- Salt and pepper to taste

Instructions:

1. Preheat the oven to 425°F (220°C).
2. Slice cauliflower heads into thick "steaks."
3. In a bowl, mix olive oil, smoked paprika, garlic powder, onion powder, salt, and pepper.
4. Brush the cauliflower steaks with the mixture.
5. Roast for 20-25 minutes until tender.

Lemon Garlic Asparagus Pasta

Ingredients:

- 8 oz pasta (use gluten-free if needed)
- 1 bunch asparagus, trimmed and cut into 2-inch pieces
- 2 tablespoons olive oil
- 2 cloves garlic, minced
- Zest and juice of 1 lemon
- Salt and pepper to taste
- Vegan Parmesan cheese for garnish (optional)

Instructions:

1. Cook pasta according to package instructions.
2. In a skillet, heat olive oil and sauté garlic until fragrant.
3. Add asparagus and cook for a few minutes until tender-crisp.
4. Toss cooked pasta with lemon zest, lemon juice, asparagus, salt, and pepper.
5. Garnish with vegan Parmesan cheese if desired.

Chapter 5: Snacks and Appetizers

When it comes to satisfying your snack cravings and wowing your guests with appetizers, you'll find a delightful assortment of options in this chapter. From the creamy goodness of guacamole to the crunch of baked zucchini chips, these recipes are not only delicious but also entirely plant-based and perfect for those looking for healthy snack alternatives.

Guacamole with Veggie Sticks

Ingredients:

- 2 ripe avocados
- 1 small onion, finely chopped
- 1 clove garlic, minced
- 1 tomato, diced
- 1 lime, juiced
- Salt and pepper to taste
- Assorted vegetable sticks for dipping (carrots, cucumbers, bell peppers)

Instructions:

1. Cut the avocados in half, remove the seeds, and scoop the flesh into a bowl.
2. Mash the avocados with a fork until creamy.
3. Stir in the chopped onion, minced garlic, diced tomato, and lime juice.
4. Season with salt and pepper to taste.
5. Serve with a platter of fresh vegetable sticks for dipping.

Salsa and Baked Tortilla Chips

Ingredients:

- 4 ripe tomatoes, diced
- 1/2 red onion, finely chopped
- 1/4 cup fresh cilantro, chopped
- 1 jalapeño pepper, seeds removed and finely chopped (adjust to your preferred spice level)
- 2 cloves garlic, minced
- Juice of 2 limes
- Salt and pepper to taste
- Whole-grain tortillas

Instructions:

1. Preheat the oven to 350°F (175°C).
2. Cut the tortillas into triangles and place them on a baking sheet.
3. Bake in the preheated oven for about 10-15 minutes or until they are crispy.
4. In a bowl, combine the diced tomatoes, chopped red onion, cilantro, jalapeño, garlic, and lime juice.
5. Season with salt and pepper to taste.
6. Serve the salsa with the baked tortilla chips.

Edamame with Sea Salt

Ingredients:

- 2 cups frozen edamame
- Sea salt to taste

Instructions:

1. Boil the edamame in a pot of water according to the package instructions.
2. Drain the edamame and sprinkle with sea salt.
3. Serve hot as a delightful and protein-packed snack.

Carrot and Cucumber Slices with Hummus

Ingredients:

- Carrots, cucumbers, or your choice of fresh veggies, sliced
- Hummus for dipping

Instructions:

1. Wash, peel, and slice the carrots, cucumbers, or any other vegetables you prefer.
2. Serve with a side of creamy hummus for dipping.

Vegan Spring Rolls

Ingredients:

- Rice paper wrappers
- Lettuce leaves
- Thin rice noodles, cooked and cooled
- Julienned carrots
- Sliced cucumber
- Fresh mint leaves
- Cooked and sliced tofu or tempeh (optional)

- Peanut dipping sauce

Instructions:

1. Soak the rice paper wrappers in warm water until pliable.
2. Lay a lettuce leaf on each wrapper and top with rice noodles, carrots, cucumber, mint leaves, and tofu or tempeh if desired.
3. Roll up the spring rolls, tucking in the sides, to enclose the filling.
4. Serve with peanut dipping sauce.

Roasted Red Pepper Hummus

Ingredients:

- 2 red bell peppers
- 1 can (15 oz) chickpeas, drained and rinsed
- 2 cloves garlic, minced
- 2 tablespoons tahini
- 2 tablespoons lemon juice
- 2 tablespoons olive oil
- Salt and pepper to taste

Instructions:

1. Preheat the oven to 450°F (230°C).
2. Roast the red bell peppers until the skin is charred and blistered. Then, peel and remove the seeds.
3. In a food processor, combine the roasted red peppers, chickpeas, garlic, tahini, lemon juice, and olive oil.
4. Process until smooth, adding salt and pepper to taste.
5. Serve with your choice of dippers.

Avocado Fries

Ingredients:

- 2 ripe avocados
- 1 cup breadcrumbs (use gluten-free if needed)
- 1 teaspoon paprika
- Salt and pepper to taste
- Cooking spray

Instructions:

1. Preheat your oven to 425°F (220°C).
2. Cut the avocados into thick slices.
3. In a bowl, combine breadcrumbs, paprika, salt, and pepper.

4. Dip each avocado slice into the breadcrumb mixture, making sure they're well coated.

5. Place the coated slices on a baking sheet, lightly spray them with cooking spray, and bake for about 15-20 minutes or until golden and crispy.

Sweet Potato Fries

Ingredients:

- 2 sweet potatoes, cut into fries
- 1 tablespoon olive oil
- 1/2 teaspoon paprika
- Salt and pepper to taste

Instructions:

1. Preheat the oven to 425°F (220°C).

2. In a bowl, toss sweet potato fries with olive oil, paprika, salt, and pepper.

3. Spread them in a single layer on a baking sheet.

4. Bake for 20-25 minutes or until they are crisp and golden.

Stuffed Mushrooms

Ingredients:

- 18 large mushrooms, cleaned and stems removed
- 1/2 cup breadcrumbs (use gluten-free if needed)
- 1/4 cup chopped onion
- 1/4 cup chopped bell pepper
- 2 cloves garlic, minced
- 1 tablespoon olive oil
- Salt and pepper to taste

Instructions:

1. Preheat your oven to 350°F (175°C).
2. In a skillet, heat olive oil and sauté the onion, bell pepper, and garlic until softened.
3. In a bowl, mix the sautéed vegetables with breadcrumbs and season with salt and pepper.
4. Fill each mushroom cap with the breadcrumb mixture.
5. Place the stuffed mushrooms on a baking sheet and bake for about 15-20 minutes or until they're tender and golden.

Quinoa-Stuffed Bell Peppers

Ingredients:

- 4 bell peppers, tops and seeds removed
- 1 cup quinoa, cooked
- 1 can (15 oz) black beans, drained and rinsed
- 1 cup corn (fresh, frozen, or canned)
- 1 cup diced tomatoes
- 1 teaspoon chili powder
- Salt and pepper to taste

Instructions:

1. Preheat your oven to 350°F (175°C).
2. In a bowl, mix the cooked quinoa, black beans, corn, diced tomatoes, chili powder, salt, and pepper.
3. Stuff each bell pepper with the quinoa mixture.
4. Place the stuffed peppers in a baking dish and bake for about 25-30 minutes or until the peppers are tender.

Vegan Onion Rings

Ingredients:

- 2 large onions, cut into rings
- 1 cup all-purpose flour (or gluten-free flour)
- 1 cup plant-based milk
- 1 cup breadcrumbs (use gluten-free if needed)
- 1 teaspoon paprika
- Salt and pepper to taste
- Cooking oil for frying

Instructions:

1. In a bowl, combine flour, plant-based milk, paprika, salt, and pepper to create a batter.
2. Dip each onion ring into the batter, allowing any excess to drip off.
3. Coat the battered onion rings with breadcrumbs.
4. Heat oil in a deep frying pan and fry the onion rings until golden brown.
5. Place them on a paper towel to remove excess oil.

Roasted Chickpeas

Ingredients:

- 2 cans (15 oz each) chickpeas, drained and rinsed
- 2 tablespoons olive oil
- 1 teaspoon paprika
- 1 teaspoon cumin
- Salt and pepper to taste

Instructions:

1. Preheat your oven to 400°F (200°C).
2. Pat the chickpeas dry with a towel to remove excess moisture.
3. In a bowl, toss the chickpeas with olive oil, paprika, cumin, salt, and pepper.
4. Spread them on a baking sheet and roast for about 25-30 minutes, or until they are crispy.

Vegan Spinach Artichoke Dip

Ingredients:

- 1 cup frozen spinach, thawed and drained
- 1 can (14 oz) artichoke hearts, drained and chopped

- 1 cup vegan cream cheese
- 1/2 cup vegan mayonnaise
- 1/2 cup vegan Parmesan cheese
- 2 cloves garlic, minced
- Salt and pepper to taste

Instructions:

1. Preheat your oven to 350°F (175°C).
2. In a mixing bowl, combine the thawed spinach, chopped artichoke hearts, vegan cream cheese, vegan mayonnaise, vegan Parmesan cheese, minced garlic, salt, and pepper.
3. Transfer the mixture to a baking dish and bake for about 25-30 minutes, or until it's bubbly and golden.

Cucumber Avocado Rolls

Ingredients:

- 2 large cucumbers
- 1 ripe avocado, mashed
- 1/4 cup red bell pepper, diced
- 1/4 cup carrot, julienned
- 1/4 cup alfalfa sprouts

- Fresh cilantro leaves
- Soy sauce or tamari for dipping

Instructions:

1. Cut the cucumbers lengthwise into thin strips using a peeler.
2. Lay out a cucumber strip, spread a thin layer of mashed avocado, and add some diced red bell pepper, julienned carrot, alfalfa sprouts, and cilantro leaves.
3. Roll up the cucumber strip like a sushi roll.
4. Serve with a side of soy sauce or tamari for dipping.

Stuffed Grape Leaves

Ingredients:

- 30-40 grape leaves (canned or fresh)
- 1 cup cooked rice
- 1/2 cup finely chopped fresh dill
- 1/4 cup lemon juice
- 1/4 cup olive oil
- Salt and pepper to taste

Instructions:

1. If using fresh grape leaves, blanch them in boiling water until they are soft. If using canned grape leaves, rinse and drain them.
2. In a bowl, mix the cooked rice, chopped dill, lemon juice, olive oil, salt, and pepper.
3. Place a grape leaf flat on a surface and add a small spoonful of the rice mixture.
4. Roll up the grape leaf, tucking in the sides, to create a stuffed grape leaf.
5. Serve chilled.

Baked Zucchini Chips

Ingredients:

- 2 zucchinis, sliced into thin rounds
- 1 cup breadcrumbs (use gluten-free if needed)
- 1/2 cup vegan Parmesan cheese
- 1 teaspoon dried oregano
- Salt and pepper to taste
- Cooking spray

Instructions:

1. Preheat your oven to 425°F (220°C).

2. In a bowl, combine breadcrumbs, vegan Parmesan cheese, dried oregano, salt, and pepper.

3. Dip each zucchini round into the breadcrumb mixture, ensuring they are well-coated.

4. Place the coated zucchini rounds on a baking sheet, lightly spray them with cooking spray, and bake for about 20-25 minutes or until they are crispy.

Vegan Bruschetta

Ingredients:

- 4-5 ripe tomatoes, diced
- 1/4 cup fresh basil, chopped
- 2 cloves garlic, minced
- 1/4 cup red onion, finely chopped
- 2 tablespoons balsamic vinegar
- Salt and pepper to taste
- Slices of whole-grain bread, toasted

Instructions:

1. In a bowl, combine diced tomatoes, fresh basil, minced garlic, chopped red onion, balsamic vinegar, salt, and pepper.

2. Spoon the mixture onto toasted whole-grain bread slices.

3. Serve as a delightful appetizer.

Vegan Nachos

Ingredients:

- Whole-grain tortilla chips
- 1 can (15 oz) black beans, drained and rinsed
- 1 cup vegan cheese, shredded
- Sliced jalapeños (optional)
- Salsa
- Guacamole

Instructions:

1. Arrange the tortilla chips on a baking sheet.

2. Sprinkle black beans and vegan cheese over the chips.

3. Add sliced jalapeños if desired.

4. Bake in a preheated oven at 350°F (175°C) until the cheese is melted.

5. Serve with salsa and guacamole for dipping.

Chapter 6: Desserts

In this chapter, we'll explore a variety of sweet treats that are not only kind to your blood sugar levels but also bursting with flavor. From fruity delights to chocolaty pleasures, these desserts are sure to satisfy your sweet tooth without compromising your health. Let's dive into these delightful recipes, each designed to bring a touch of sweetness into your life.

Banana Ice Cream

Ingredients:

- 2 ripe bananas, sliced and frozen
- 1 teaspoon vanilla extract (optional)

Instructions:

1. Place the frozen banana slices in a food processor.
2. Add vanilla extract if desired.
3. Blend until smooth and creamy, resembling ice cream.
4. Serve immediately or freeze for a firmer texture.

Vegan Chocolate Avocado Mousse

Ingredients:

- 2 ripe avocados
- 1/4 cup cocoa powder
- 1/4 cup maple syrup
- 1 teaspoon vanilla extract

Instructions:

1. Scoop the flesh from the avocados into a food processor.
2. Add cocoa powder, maple syrup, and vanilla extract.
3. Blend until smooth and creamy.
4. Chill in the refrigerator before serving.

Berry Parfait

Ingredients:

- 1 cup mixed berries (strawberries, blueberries, raspberries)
- 1 cup dairy-free yogurt
- 1/4 cup granola (sugar-free)

Instructions:

1. In a glass or bowl, layer the berries and yogurt.
2. Top with granola.
3. Repeat the layers.
4. Serve immediately for a refreshing dessert.

Coconut Bliss Balls

Ingredients:

- 1 cup shredded coconut
- 1/2 cup almond flour
- 1/4 cup coconut oil
- 2 tablespoons maple syrup
- 1 teaspoon vanilla extract

Instructions:

1. In a bowl, mix all ingredients until well combined.
2. Roll the mixture into small balls.
3. Chill in the refrigerator to set.
4. Enjoy as a quick energy boost.

Chia Seed Pudding with Berries

Ingredients:

- 3 tablespoons chia seeds
- 1 cup unsweetened almond milk
- 1 tablespoon maple syrup
- 1/2 cup mixed berries

Instructions:

1. Mix chia seeds, almond milk, and maple syrup in a jar.
2. Stir well and refrigerate overnight.
3. In the morning, top with mixed berries.
4. A healthy and filling dessert is ready to enjoy.

Vegan Chocolate Chip Cookies

Ingredients:

- 1 cup almond flour
- 1/4 cup coconut oil
- 1/4 cup maple syrup
- 1/2 teaspoon baking soda
- 1/4 cup dairy-free chocolate chips

Instructions:

1. Preheat the oven to 350°F (175°C).

2. In a bowl, mix almond flour, coconut oil, maple syrup, and baking soda.

3. Fold in chocolate chips.

4. Drop spoonfuls of dough onto a baking sheet.

5. Bake for 12-15 minutes until golden brown.

Almond Joy Energy Bites

Ingredients:

- 1 cup rolled oats
- 1/2 cup almond butter
- 1/4 cup shredded coconut
- 1/4 cup chopped almonds
- 2 tablespoons cocoa powder
- 2 tablespoons maple syrup

Instructions:

1. In a bowl, combine oats, almond butter, shredded coconut, chopped almonds, cocoa powder, and maple syrup.

2. Roll the mixture into bite-sized balls.

3. Chill in the refrigerator before serving.

Vegan Apple Crisp

Ingredients:

- 4 cups sliced apples
- 1/2 cup rolled oats
- 1/4 cup almond flour
- 1/4 cup maple syrup
- 1/4 cup coconut oil
- 1/2 teaspoon cinnamon

Instructions:

1. Preheat the oven to 350°F (175°C).
2. In a bowl, mix oats, almond flour, maple syrup, coconut oil, and cinnamon.
3. Layer sliced apples in a baking dish.
4. Top with the oat mixture.
5. Bake for 30-35 minutes until golden and bubbly.

Chocolate-Dipped Strawberries

Ingredients:

- 12 fresh strawberries
- 1/4 cup dairy-free chocolate chips

Instructions:

1. Melt the chocolate chips in a microwave-safe bowl.
2. Dip each strawberry into the melted chocolate.
3. Place on a tray lined with parchment paper.
4. Let them cool and harden.

Cinnamon Baked Apples

Ingredients:

- 4 apples, cored and sliced
- 1 teaspoon ground cinnamon
- 2 tablespoons maple syrup
- 1/4 cup chopped walnuts (optional)

Instructions:

1. Preheat the oven to 350°F (175°C).

2. Toss the apple slices with cinnamon and maple syrup.

3. Spread them in a baking dish.

4. If desired, sprinkle chopped walnuts on top.

5. Bake for 25-30 minutes until apples are tender and fragrant.

Vegan Rice Pudding

Ingredients:

- 1 cup cooked rice
- 2 cups unsweetened almond milk
- 1/4 cup raisins
- 1/4 cup maple syrup
- 1 teaspoon vanilla extract
- 1/2 teaspoon ground cinnamon

Instructions:

1. In a saucepan, combine rice, almond milk, raisins, maple syrup, vanilla extract, and cinnamon.

2. Cook over low heat, stirring occasionally, until it thickens.

3. Serve warm or chilled.

Mango Sorbet

Ingredients:

- 2 cups frozen mango chunks
- 1/4 cup coconut milk
- 2 tablespoons lime juice
- 2 tablespoons agave nectar

Instructions:

1. Blend frozen mango, coconut milk, lime juice, and agave nectar until smooth.
2. Pour into a container and freeze until firm.
3. Scoop and enjoy a tropical delight.

Vegan Pumpkin Pie

Ingredients:

- 1 vegan pie crust
- 1 1/2 cups canned pumpkin
- 1/2 cup coconut milk
- 1/2 cup maple syrup
- 1 teaspoon pumpkin spice
- 1/2 teaspoon cinnamon

Instructions:

1. Preheat the oven to 350°F (175°C).
2. In a bowl, mix pumpkin, coconut milk, maple syrup, pumpkin spice, and cinnamon.
3. Pour the mixture into the pie crust.
4. Bake for 40-45 minutes until the filling is set.
5. Allow it to cool before serving.

Chocolate Zucchini Brownies

Ingredients:

- 1 cup shredded zucchini
- 1/4 cup cocoa powder
- 1/2 cup almond flour
- 1/4 cup maple syrup
- 1/4 cup dairy-free chocolate chips

Instructions:

1. Preheat the oven to 350°F (175°C).
2. In a bowl, combine zucchini, cocoa powder, almond flour, maple syrup, and chocolate chips.
3. Spread the mixture in a baking dish.
4. Bake for 25-30 minutes until brownies are set.

Lemon Blueberry Bars

Ingredients:

- 1 cup almond flour
- 1/4 cup coconut oil
- 1/4 cup maple syrup
- 1 cup fresh blueberries
- Zest and juice of 1 lemon

Instructions:

1. Preheat the oven to 350°F (175°C).
2. In a bowl, mix almond flour, coconut oil, and maple syrup.
3. Press the mixture into a baking dish.
4. Sprinkle blueberries, lemon zest, and lemon juice on top.
5. Bake for 20-25 minutes until golden brown.

Vegan Cheesecake

Ingredients:

- 1 cup cashews (soaked and drained)
- 1/4 cup coconut oil

- 1/4 cup maple syrup
- 1/4 cup lemon juice
- 1 teaspoon vanilla extract

Instructions:

1. Blend soaked cashews, coconut oil, maple syrup, lemon juice, and vanilla extract until smooth.
2. Pour the mixture into a pie crust and refrigerate until set.

Berry Sorbet

Ingredients:

- 2 cups mixed berries (strawberries, blueberries, raspberries)
- 1/4 cup agave nectar
- 1 tablespoon lemon juice

Instructions:

1. Blend mixed berries, agave nectar, and lemon juice until smooth.
2. Freeze the mixture until firm.
3. Scoop and enjoy a refreshing treat.

Pistachio Date Bites

Ingredients:

- 1 cup dates
- 1/2 cup shelled pistachios
- 1/4 cup shredded coconut

Instructions:

1. In a food processor, blend dates and pistachios until the mixture sticks together.
2. Roll into small bites and coat with shredded coconut.

CONCLUSION

As we come to the end of this journey through the world of diabetic-friendly plant-based recipes, it's essential to reflect on the incredible transformation you've experienced. Your commitment to embracing a healthier lifestyle is commendable, and your dedication to managing diabetes through plant-based choices has set you on a path to long-lasting well-being.

In this concluding chapter, we'd like to offer some heartfelt guidance to ensure your success in maintaining this newfound way of life. Let's explore a few essential points that can help you stay on track and continue to savor the benefits of this dietary shift.

Tips for Sustaining a Diabetic-Friendly Plant-Based Lifestyle:

1. **Stay Informed:** Knowledge is power, so continue to educate yourself about the latest developments in

plant-based nutrition and diabetes management. This will empower you to make informed choices and adapt to any changes that may arise.

2. **Embrace Variety:** Don't be afraid to experiment with new ingredients and flavors. Variety in your diet not only keeps things exciting but also ensures that you're getting a wide range of essential nutrients.

3. **Plan and Prep:** Success often hinges on preparation. Take the time to plan your meals and snacks, making it easier to stick to your dietary goals. Preparing larger batches of your favorite recipes can save you time during busy days.

4. **Lean on Support:** Share your journey with family and friends, as their support can make a significant difference. Additionally, there are various online communities and support groups dedicated to plant-based living and diabetes management.

5. **Listen to Your Body**: Every individual is unique, and what works for one person might not work for another. Pay attention to how your body responds to different foods and adjust your choices accordingly.

6. **Monitor Your Progress:** Regularly monitor your blood sugar levels and other health indicators. This will help you track your progress and make necessary adjustments to your dietary and lifestyle choices.

ACKNOWLEDGMENTS

This journey wouldn't have been possible without the support of countless individuals who contributed their expertise and passion to this cookbook. We extend our gratitude to the chefs, nutritionists, and healthcare professionals who have generously shared their knowledge and recipes.

In closing, we want to express our heartfelt wishes for your continued success in managing diabetes and enjoying the delicious, wholesome meals that this cookbook has to offer. Your commitment to your well-being is truly inspiring, and we hope these recipes have made a positive impact on your life.

As you move forward, remember that your health is a precious gift, and your choices play a pivotal role in preserving it. May your journey be filled with good health, delicious food, and the joy of sharing these experiences with loved ones. Thank you for being a part of our plant-based community, and here's to a vibrant, fulfilling, and diabetes-manageable future.